# A Boy
# Named
# Vinny

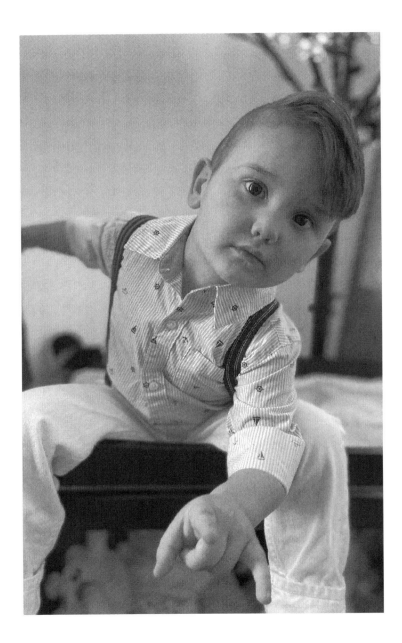

ANGELA ACKER

# A Boy Named Vinny

Holistic, non-invasive ways to give your autistic child a more sustainable life

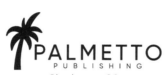

Charleston, SC
www.PalmettoPublishing.com

*A Boy Named Vinny*

Copyright © 2022 by Angela Acker

First Edition

Paperback ISBN: 979-8-88590-299-1
eBook ISBN: 979-8-88590-300-4

# For My Son:

. . .

*I dislike it when you look at me.*

*I dislike it when you stare.*

*If you knew how loud noises affect me,*
*would you really care?*

*My mommy tries to protect me from all that bothers me.*
*But why can't the world also do that for me?*

*We need more protectors in every shape and form. We*
*need autism to not be disregarded and instead*
*be reformed.*

*Bring sensory rooms to venues and try dimming down*
*the lights. Let these kids know we care about their fights.*

*Every day they face successfully is another battle won,*
*let's give these kids a fighting chance*
*instead of not having one.*

. . .

## With Love,
## Mommy

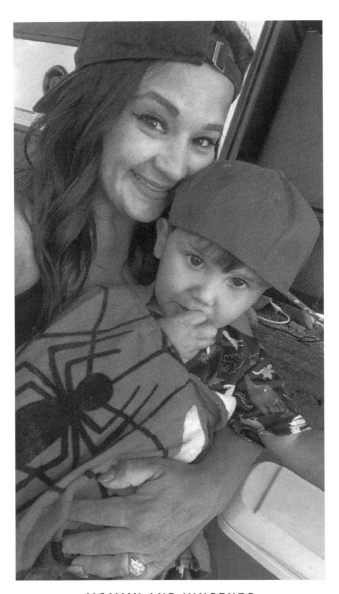

MOMMY AND VINCENZO

# Table of Contents

# Introduction

Hello, my name is Angela and my husband's name is Bradley, and we are the proud parents of Vincenzo Roman. Vincenzo was created with love and science, and for that, we are eternally grateful. We thought the hardest part would be conceiving Vincenzo, due to struggling with infertility, but we were completely wrong. The first years to come would be one of the hardest years we would ever have to face. Vincenzo was born neurotypical, hitting milestones, and becoming his own person until something happened and my son's light was gone, and Vincenzo drifted far away from me. We never thought we would be able to share his story or even speak about his diagnosis, but we know none of this would define him. We thought to ourselves if we can help at least one child with the same disorder then sharing his story would make his journey worthwhile.

On January 8th, 2021, Vincenzo was diagnosed with level 2 or moderate autism. His T-score was equivalent to 50, demonstrating severe symptoms of autism spectrum disorder. Vinny was completely nonverbal, ear covering in response to certain noises; he hurt himself, screamed, fell when attempting to walk, mouthed everything he came into contact with, ran in circles, breath-holding episodes, flapped hands, stared off into space, and the worst thing that happened he disconnected himself from everyone. I want you to imagine being able to hold your baby, feed them a bottle, and rock them to sleep and suddenly at their age of fifteen months, all of that changed. After all the pain I went through to conceive and carry him for nine months, my baby would no longer let me do the things I once did for him when he was an infant. He did not prefer me; he wanted my husband, and that was his person. Vincenzo was no longer his happy-go-lucky self, instead, he drifted off to a place I could not reach and I did not know what to do. I never want any parent to go through what my family had to. Although, one in forty-four children are being diagnosed with autism, and that number is higher in boys.

During this time, we were also going through the coronavirus pandemic, and as a result, after being diagnosed with moderate autism, my son was left with Zoom speech once a week for thirty minutes, and that was it. Talk about the worst time when something like this can happen. When people are scared to be around others, how would we help my baby? We will tell you what we did and how much it helped our child immensely. What we are going to share with you may help a family member, a friend, a neighbor, or a coworker, and to me, that is paying it forward. God gave me Vinny for a reason and what happened to him serves a much higher purpose. Parents need to stick together and share their knowledge to help each other. It is not about who or what to blame for his autism—to me, it was just moving forward. That is the importance of moving forward and never looking back to that dark stage in our life again. This story is very personal, and I want you to know it took much courage to share this. You will not find cited sources or quotations in this book; this is raw emotion of a mother and father's love for their child.

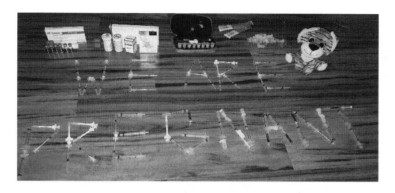

**PREGNANCY ANNOUNCEMENT FOR VINCENZO**

# CHAPTER 1

# The Start of Our Journey

never thought in my wildest dreams that I would ever be told my child has autism. As you know, autism is a life-long diagnosis. The day I found out my son had autism was the day I realized I would need to fight with all my might to figure out what happened to my son. My child was walking by age eleven months, babbling all of the time, and even saying certain words, to absolutely nothing. If this is genetic autism then why would he suddenly change instead of always being in this state? My child was not there. This is a feeling or pain that is unexplainable, unbearable, and hopefully, whoever is reading this will never have to go through it. I hope that if you do know someone who is going through this, you are there for them, and I hope you support them.

Let us rewind a bit to where this all began—when my oldest son Luciano asked for a sibling, and I told him to be patient. Luciano was three years old at the time. By the time he was five, we were still unable to conceive and realized we needed to explore other options. The infertility specialist we met with stated we will not be able to conceive naturally due to a male factor and female factor. We were not ready to give up. Birth of Luciano took seven years and multiple rounds of Clomid until we conceived our miracle, so we were not giving up this easy and proceeded with IVF. From start to finish, IVF took a lot of time and money, and it took a toll on my health. From the endless injections, multiple sonograms, and becoming bedridden from my egg retrieval, I was still not ready to give up. I will never forget the day we implanted our very first embryo (which happens to be my third son Alfonso's date of birth. Funny how things work out on God's time). I remember holding hands with my husband and our fertility specialist, and we said a prayer for successful implantation. That night was followed by a pizza date and a warm hug from my five-year-old once we got home. He said, "Mommy, did we get our baby?" I answered, "We will wait and see what God has in store for us." I just remember feeling pregnant right away; after multiple losses, I was finally pregnant. I called my fertility specialist and requested an hCG blood draw. She stated it was exceedingly early and may not be accurate but if it would put my nerves at ease, she will order one. Once I took the blood test, I remember just feeling so happy inside. This time around, I was not nervous about losing the baby; I just felt like this was it for us. After stalking my patient portal for multiple hours, I finally saw what I was waiting for; we finally achieved our positive pregnancy test. My hCG level was 9.5 mIU/mL and I was carrying our little bundle of joy. Of course, I had to call my best friend and inform her that we would need a onesie created with a design on the onesie saying "Anything over 5 is considered pregnant and mine is 9.5." I picked up the onesie on my way home from work and gave the box to my husband and Luciano. I will never forget my husband's reaction; he said "Babe, are you serious?" Then he looked at Luciano and said, "We are having a baby!" Everyone thought I should not have told my son so early that we were having a baby, but to me, I never thought once that I would lose my baby. I knew that God would protect our little one and keep him safe.

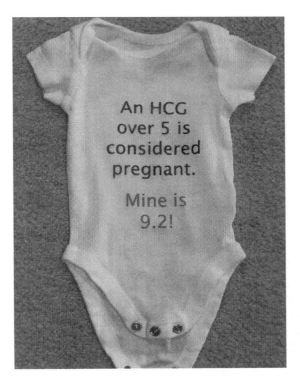

**HOW I ANNOUNCED THE PREGNANCY TO BRAD AND LUCIANO**

I always say, "Do what works for you and don't judge others for what they do." Everyone does things differently with their kids and their lives, and all you can do is what is best for your family and your situation. It took me a while to learn that. I did not understand why people took their fertility for granted. Having a baby through IVF is not just mentally draining; it is emotionally and physically draining as well. It may take a toll on your mind, body, health, and marriage. The biggest benefit of IVF to me was not only the ability to have a baby but we also were able to have each embryo genetically tested. Vincenzo Roman was graded AAA embryo, meaning he was genetically perfect, and that's the embryo we started with. I still remember the fertility specialist saying "You and your husband make beautiful embryos; your problem is just implantation, and we will help you with that." On December 16th, 2017, Vincenzo Roman Acker was implanted in my uterus—the day I will never forget. Our child was made with love and science. I thought the hard part was over; however, I was wrong, very wrong. The hardest part was yet to come.

# CHAPTER 2

# Vincenzo's Birth

O n August 24, 2018, I walked into the hospital at 5:30 am for our scheduled C-section. I just remember feeling happy and scared. My first C-section was emergent due to my first son having breathing issues in the womb. We almost lost our first child due to an adverse reaction to Pitocin. As they prepped me for my spinal anesthetic, I realized that I could still feel my feet, and the spinal injection was not working. The resident checked with the anesthesiologist and told the doctor I was still able to feel my feet. The doctor informed the resident that they missed my spine and had to do it again. At this point, I felt so incredibly ill, with double the amount of anesthesia followed by morphine to numb the pain. I was in the OR for a total of three hours, maybe a little longer give or take, but what I do remember is profusely vomiting later due to the excessive amount of morphine. I could not hold Vinny for long after he was born because I was extremely sick. Thankfully, my husband was able to do skin to skin with him and give him all the love I physically could not give because my body would not let me.

Just few hours after he was born, the nurse came in and administered the hepatitis B vaccine. She kept insisting it was the best for the baby, and it was the safest for the baby, and here I was thinking, *I am a health-care professional myself; this must be okay for our baby.* I mean, why wouldn't vaccines be 100 percent safe for babies? I wish I had asked myself those questions. I wish I would have done my due diligence and read more articles regarding this vaccine and many others. However, with a healthy five-year-old at the time who was fully vaccinated, I felt and thought I should do the same with my new baby as I have done with my oldest. I have now at this point worked for the health-care system for ten years, and I have trusted every doctor I have met as well as my pediatrician.

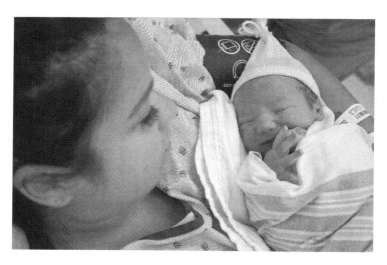

MOMMY & VINCENZO

Vinny was my biggest baby. He was seven pounds seven ounces and twenty inches long. I lost my father at an incredibly young age, and all I remember is my husband saying "Babe, he looks just like your father. I can't believe it; he looks just like him." I remember looking over and just crying because I saw my father in this baby. My world stopped for a minute, and I could not believe after so many injections, ultrasounds, blood work, and tears, my baby was here. I knew that very moment our bond would be everlasting.

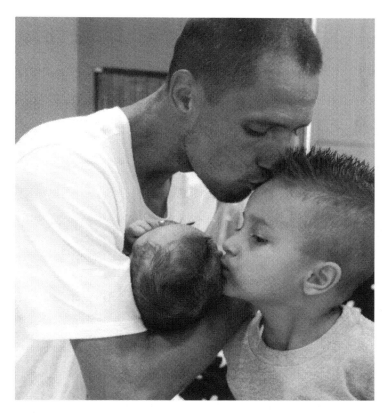

**DADDY, LUCIANO & VINCENZO**

Once we had Vincenzo, I thought it was time for a new pediatrician. Before this pediatrician, we were with a much larger pediatric group, and I did not feel comfortable with multiple providers treating my children and giving multiple, different medical opinions on each visit. Our new pediatric office consisted of two physicians and that made me feel more comfortable. Our first visit was very educational and informative. One of the very first questions was, "Did he get his hepatitis B vaccine?" I replied, "Yes, he did in the hospital," and before I could ask why do they need a vaccine this soon after birth, I was directed to a different subject. I just remember being super tired and sore. My incision site was still very raw and just carrying the baby was a lot of pain for me, but I did not care—anything for my babies. From that appointment until Vinny was fifteen months of age, he was amazing us with achieving milestones, with his smiles, and with his laughter. I absolutely love taking pictures and videos of my children, my mom refers to me as the "paparazzi". I had not had a baby in over five years, so obsessing over every moment spent with him, just like I did with my oldest. I am happy I was able to do that because this solidifies all my truth about what happened to my son after we left his fifteen-month wellness visit. My son went from hitting milestones, and displaying eye contact, to absolutely nothing. At fifteen months old, Vinny was drifting further and further from his mommy, daddy, and brother. Vinny chose to be alone, and he no longer wanted or craved affection. Vinny was in his own little world and stayed that way for quite some time.

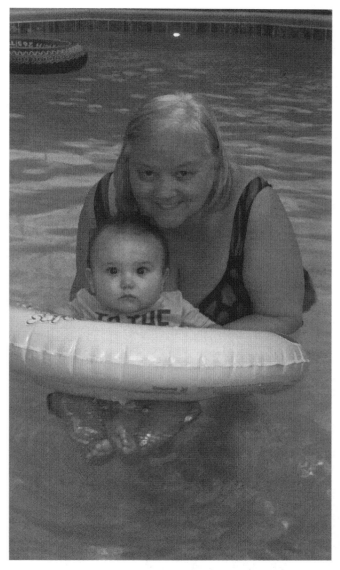

VINNY AT EIGHT MONTHS OLD WITH GRANDMA

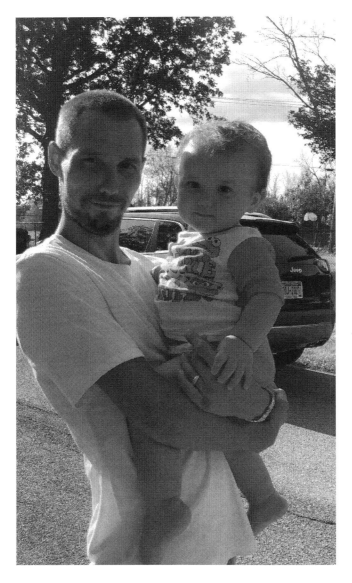

VINNY AT THIRTEEN MONTHS OLD.

# CHAPTER 3:

# Fifteen-Month Wellness Visit

Vinny hit many milestones, much earlier than my oldest did. I remember joking around calling him my grade A embryo and that is why he was doing things so fast. At four months old, Vinny would try to sit up on his boppy chair; at six months, he was crawling and babbling. He was standing at ten months and walking by eleven months and displayed amazing balance. Everything just seemed like it was easy for him. I even remember, at four weeks old, he was trying to grab and hold his own bottle. I also remember, at eleven months old, placing him on his potty chair and telling him to pee-pee on the potty, and he looked at me, then looked down, and then stood up, and long behold, there were a few drops of pee in his potty seat. We just started screaming in joy, "Vinny, good job! You went pee-pee on the potty." I remember just thinking to myself, *What is this kid? A baby genius?*

Vinny was generally a healthy baby. He also loved eating healthy. He craved fruits and vegetables and never really wanted or chose to eat things that were not the best for him. He did experience a few colds here and there, but I chalked that up to school germs from his older brother. I remember going to his fifteen-month appointment and telling the doctor about his birthday party and how he was looking at everyone and he loved everyone singing to him. He generally loved being around everyone and everything. At this point, I was not worried about my child having a developmental disability when he was reaching milestones before most children would. The pediatrician said, "Well, today we will be administering his fifteen-month vaccines, and lucky for you, they combined the vaccines and instead separate needle sticks, he will only have one. Today, Vincenzo will receive his MMRV vaccine."

- This is when I wish I would have paused and asked, "Are we able to separate them? Will there be double the number of metals in these vaccines? How common are adverse reactions and could this vaccine cause a febrile seizure? Can we maybe delay this vaccine until he is a little bit bigger or when his brain is fully developed?" After all, they do not want you to think something like this could happen. I understand it does not happen to every child, but it happened to mine. All I can say is once you know better, you do better. I now ask those questions when I am at the doctor's office and I make sure I voice all of my concerns. I am not here to bash pediatricians. I absolutely love my current pediatrician and I have so much profound respect for her. Every wellness visit, we are able to ask questions without feeling uncomfortable for asking those questions. Every decision we make for our children can affect them for days or years from now, so it's very important to research and ask questions.

# CHAPTER 4:

# The Night of Vinny's Reaction

The very next day of his appointment was Thanksgiving, and the pediatrician said, "Why don't you give this little guy some Motrin or Tylenol if he feels uncomfortable, he should be okay and we will see you at his next wellness visit." That day we came home and placed Vinny in his crib. I remember that night as if it were yesterday. It is the day that changed my son's life. I remember the movie that was playing, the pajamas Vinny was wearing, and everything following that. I struggle to remember some things in my life, but this incident I will never forget.

Around midnight, Vincenzo woke up with a blood-curdling scream. We immediately knew something was wrong and took him out of his crib and placed him into the bed with us. As minutes passed by, he started crying inconsolably and my mommy intuition said something was not right here. At this point, he started burning up and the fever was at 103, and I was extremely concerned. This did not happen with my oldest, and I knew something was horribly wrong. I phoned the pediatrician on call and, of course, with it being the day before the holiday, I ended up speaking with a pediatrician who did not know my child by any means. She observed his electronic medical record and gave me her medical opinion. She asked a few questions and then told me she did not think it was an adverse reaction to the vaccine as Vinny was not having a seizure; however, if we could not get him to stop crying or if the fever persisted, I was told to bring him into this nearest hospital. She insisted this could not be a reaction to the vaccine but his body showed it was responding to the vaccine. That night, I did not sleep. I remember googling articles about MMRV combo vaccines and their adverse reactions. A few of the parent blogs I read sounded just like the experience we were having but I trusted science, and I trusted our pediatrician.

The very next day was Thanksgiving Day and Vinny was still not the same. He started banging his head on his crib rail and crying and whining for a reason we did not understand at the time. At this point, I was thinking he was fussy from the vaccine and hopefully, soon we could put this behind us. When we got together with the family, I told them that Vinny was having a reaction to the vaccines and was not himself. I kid you not, as soon as my mother went to pick up her grandson, he bucked back and started crying. My mother did try to warn me about vaccines; however, I did not want to believe her. Again, who would think this could happen? Vinny did not want to be touched by anyone, and no one could feed him at this point. He wanted to be alone or with my husband, and this continued and progressed quickly. What was happening to our son? It was very disappointing that our pediatrician did not follow up with us after my phone call to the on-call pediatrician. However, this is no longer about looking back but moving forward to heal my son. I don't hold any hate towards that physician. At the end of the day, I made the decision to have this vaccine administered to my child.

# CHAPTER 5

# Regression

Within the next few months, Vinny started spiraling. I could not take a picture or video of him. He lost complete eye contact, started headbanging, holding his breath until he turned blue, running in circles, flapping hands, and mouthing absolutely everything under the sun that warranted autism. He would also hold a phone directly to his ear when he really enjoyed something and that was a new behavior. Any time he was in his crib, he would choose to do handstand because it felt satisfying to him to be upside down. Another huge change was Vinny kept losing his balance and he would fall almost every day. I remember specifically telling our pediatrician how concerned I was and even questioned if he should be in a helmet. At this time, the pediatrician thought it was not necessary.

Each day was a different experience and it just created so much anxiety within the household because we did not know what was going on with our baby. Immediately following the vaccine reaction, Vinny started pulling on his ears, slapping his ears, and covering his ears, if noises became too much. I brought Vinny in three more times for his ears, and they simply said he had no ear infection and maybe he was pulling on his ears as a reaction from teething and having molars come in. There were many trips to urgent care for what we thought were the start of ear infections. I trusted information that was given to us and proceeded with taking care of my son. However, the very last trip to urgent care really put things into perspective. Vinny was covering ears the entire time, and the physician said, "His ears are clear and it may be time to have him evaluated for autism." I cried on the way home. My youngest sister was with me at the time and saw the pain in my eyes. She said, "It's okay sissy; Vinny will be okay. You are his mom and you are a good mom."

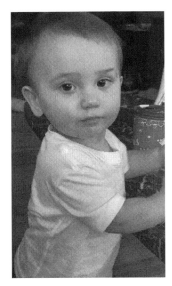 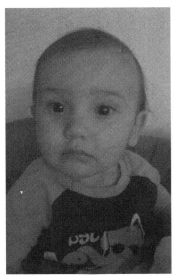

THE PICTURES ON THE LEFT AND RIGHT ARE TAKEN NOT EVEN ONE MONTH APART, AFTER HIS REACTION, AND HIS LOOK IS COMPLETELY DIFFERENT. HE WAS NOT EVEN SIXTEEN MONTHS OLD YET.

By the time Vinny was eighteen months old, I was fully a stay-at-home mom due to an unexpected natural pregnancy, and that is when all the red flags started showing. I was currently six months post-partum, pregnant again, and losing my other child to something that was beyond my control. Our son was eighteen months old, completely nonverbal, running in circles, sad, disengaged, and lost. I cannot explain this to you without showing pictures that I have but my son looked lost and disengaged. His physical appearance changed. His skin became paler, his eyes became duller, and he would no longer answer when someone would call his name. The sparkle in his eyes was gone and he was not himself. Vincenzo would no longer look at the camera; our once smiling baby would not smile or even look at me. He was so disengaged at this point he did not want to be held or touched by anyone other than his father, which took a piece of my heart and soul. I phoned my pediatrician because I was worried about his speech and disengagement. He stated that all kids are different and that I should not compare children. Vinny was always ahead with milestones and he would do it when he was ready. He said we would revisit this issue at his twenty-four-month visit. At this point, I was completely disappointed and disgusted with how my concerns were disregarded.

New behaviors were starting every single day. Vinny started purposely placing his leg in the rails of his crib and would purposely get it stuck so that he would hurt himself, along with almost passing out from a breathing spell. He would also obsess with sticking foreign objects in his ear. One evening he was standing in front of the tv in my bedroom in a daze, while chewing on one of my diamond earrings. That evening I also found a popcorn kernel in his ear. I screamed downstairs to my husband to come up and when he did, I just started crying and I told him there is something wrong our baby. Scary right? This is not normal; I know this is not normal so why am I being disregarded? Our life continued like that for well over a year.

My mommy intuition said, *No it is something more, and I am going to call Early Intervention and schedule an evaluation myself.* No one can advocate more than you; you are his parent and you are his voice. To this day, I am so happy we made that decision. I think to myself had I never made the call, Vinny would be even further behind because of the pandemic and everything else going on; it was taking months to get on board. I cannot reiterate how important it is to get the ball rolling, even if it means on your own! Never let anyone disregard your concerns when it comes to your baby.

# CHAPTER 6:

# Early Intervention

Vinny was around twenty-three months old when he was finally able to be evaluated by Early Intervention via Zoom, due to the coronavirus pandemic. The results were hard to take in but I knew deep down he was delayed with speech. His score from Early Intervention was severely low and his speech development was the same as a six-month-old's. Yes, let me repeat that to you: my child who was going to be two years old was only at a six-month-old speech development. My child who was saying words, walking before his first birthday, and even trying to be potty-trained at one year old was now further behind than we started. Imagine that feeling? It is a feeling I cannot explain to you. I cannot explain watching my younger son surpass my middle son. I could not believe that my twenty-three-month-old son was only at six months of age for speech development. The only change that we experienced with Vinny was the reaction to the combination vaccine. They stated they wanted to start him on once-a-week speech therapy via zoom, and see how things progressed. They also said he displayed other concerning behaviors but nothing at this time was revealed other than speech delay. Again, this was a twenty-three-month-old boy who was speaking at six months of age and only was allowed one session per week at thirty minutes for speech therapy.

The speech pathologist and I have become remarkably close over time. She was very empathetic, and always cared to check on us. She genuinely cares about special-needs children, and that is extremely hard to find these days. She always went the extra mile. There were many sessions of myself running around chasing him with the iPad and trying to get him to focus on his therapy. There were days I would cry to her and tell her something was going on with my son. I told her something had changed in him since that day of his reaction, and instead of getting better, Vinny started regressing more.

At this point, he no longer wanted sippy cups but only bottles; he wanted only diapers and no longer wanted to be potty trained, and he had multiple breathing holding spells a day.

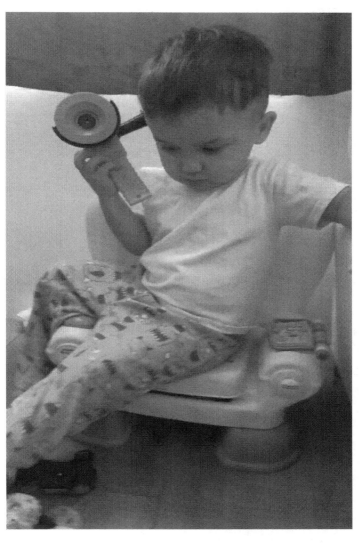

OUR LITTLE BOY WAS SO LOST; HE OFTEN
HELD THINGS UP TO HIS EAR THAT
WERE LOUD. HE OFTEN WAS ALONE.

One day, we were completing therapy and we wanted to try to demonstrate symbolic play. A big sign of autism is the child lacking symbolic play because their brain does not understand that. The speech pathologist suggested that we fill a bowl of soapy water and proceed to give Vinny his PJ Mask characters. What we thought he would do is pretend to wash them or play with them in the water. Vinny did not do any of those things; instead, he picked up the bowl of water and started drinking the water without making a face, and gagging. He simply acted as if this was normal behavior to drink soapy water. After the session ended, our speech pathologist stated it would be a good idea to request a developmental evaluation for Vinny and screen for autism. She said she observed some things with Vinny that were concerning and she agreed that he also showed signs of autism. She proceeded with sending the referral to my pediatrician and Early Intervention.

I have always felt in my heart that Vinny was special and not like my other boys. I could not ignore the signs, the breath-holding spells, him covering his ears, him sticking foreign objects in his ears, the screaming, the falling, the running in circles, and him wanting nothing to do with anyone. How much longer would this go on before we had a diagnosis? I understand pediatricians do not want to diagnose early or misdiagnose, but I wish someone listened to me when I was first coming to the office with concerns regarding Vinny. I knew at sixteen months old, my child was developing autism, and this here was the key component to trying to heal him as quickly as possible, as his brain was still developing. By the age of five, it is much harder to try to reverse symptoms of ASD. Our goal was to provide Vinny a life without so many challenges.

Multiple family members and friends would come to the house and he would not acknowledge them. Vinny was now in his own little world. I cannot imagine how he felt or what he was thinking: *Why can't I express love for others? What happened to me?* Think of how many people take the ability to speak for granted. One thing I will tell you from personal experience is that special-needs children show you life in different light; they will humble you and make you realize there is more to life than you realize.

CHAPTER 7:

# Evaluation Day

One thing that is hard to deal with during this process is how long everything takes. Evaluations takes months and sometimes up to a year to be seen. It took us four months to get an appointment at the autism center located in our hometown and took another three weeks after the evaluation to get the results. The only advice I can give regarding the waiting issue is, fill out the paperwork that day and instead of mailing it back, bring it back in person. That seemed to help a bit. On 12/21/2020, Vinny, my husband, and I entered the Robert Warner Institute. I carried Vinny's journal and was prepared to let them know exactly what was going on. I also had many videos of him before and after his adverse reaction and was able to let them observe the regression. One bit of advice I can give you is to record everything—pictures and videos of milestones. That day, he had multiple testing done and they said they would give us the results on 1/13/21, which seemed ridiculous to me. I will tell you why momentarily I feel this way. At the time of making this appointment, I knew in my heart regardless that I wanted a second opinion. If this diagnosis was going to be a permanent one without a cure then I wanted two developmental pediatricians telling me that. The University of Rochester Medical Center would give us a second opinion as well as perform the evaluation and give us the results right after the evaluation.

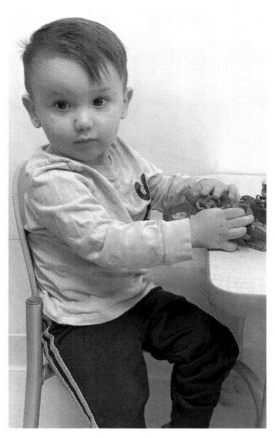

**EVALUATION DAY**

On January 8, 2021, Vincenzo had his evaluation via Zoom with URMC. At the end of the evaluation, we spoke with the physician and my phone was in my hand that was shaking when she gave us the news that Vinny had moderate autism with significant speech delay. After she stated this news, I dropped the phone and just started crying hysterically. I do not know what upset me more—the fact that my fears were confirmed or the fact that he has Autism and there is no cure for that. She did say that his motor skills were amazing and appropriate for his age, yet I told her before this, he was even doing more. She confirmed this is a form of regressive autism.

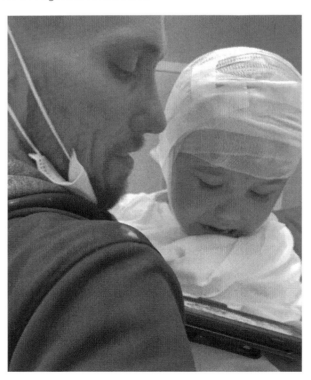

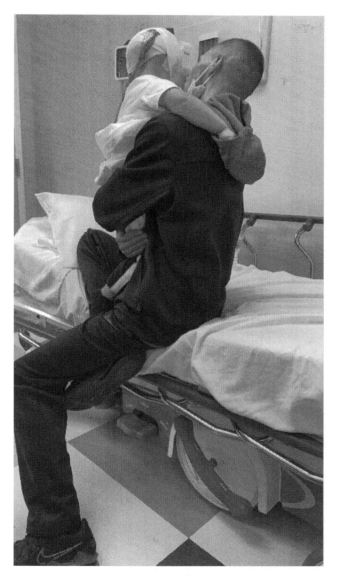

VINNY'S EEG APPOINTMENT

I kept thinking to myself, *What if he cannot ever learn to use his words? Who will be his voice when I am not here? Who is going to take care of him when I am not here too?* All of this brought me into a weird frame of mind and I started becoming more anxious and depressed than ever. I had a one-month-old infant at home, I was going through post-partum, and I was being informed that my two-year-old had autism. It was one hit after the next. I am sure a lot of people witnessed this change in me but no one ever brought it up, because no one knew what to say. What can someone say, if you genuinely think about it? That I know how you feel? Do you? Do you have a child with a permanent disability? Or do you have a child who regressed this quickly after one wellness visit?

| Standard Severity Scores | HF Severity Scores | Diagnostic Hypothesis |
|---|---|---|
| Minimal to no symptoms of ASD | Minimal to no symptoms of ASD | Nonautistic |
| 15-29.5 | 15-27.5 | |
| for ages 13+: 15-27.5 | | |
| Mild to moderate symptoms of ASD | Mild to moderate symptoms of ASD | Autism Spectrum |
| 30-36.5 | 28-33.5 | |
| for ages 13+: 28-34.5 | | |
| Severe Symptoms of ASD | Severe Symptoms of ASD | Autism Spectrum |
| 37+ | 34+ | |
| for ages 13+: 35+ | | |

The total Raw Score was 38, which falls in the range consistent with severe symptoms of ASD range. A T-score was derived, where the average scores for individuals with autism spectrum disorder fall between 45 and 54. Higher scores are indicative of higher levels of autism related symptoms compared to others with an autism spectrum disorder diagnosis. Vincenzo's T-score was: 50, indicating autism spectrum disorder.

**VINCENZO'S T-SCORE RESULTS**

CHAPTER 8:

# Meeting Our Healer

I will never forget the day we met our healer. His name is Jimmy Scaringi and he's the amazing, prestigious owner of Synergy Nutrition & Wellness located in our local town. Our healer was brought into our lives by the Casey's, who previously took their son to Synergy. The Casey's have brought so much love and joy into our lives and we are forever grateful for this relationship. To this day, we have this connection, and it is such an effortless friendship. Sometimes it is easier to have friendships with people who know exactly what you are going through and fully support your journey.

On December 28th, 2020, we walked into Jimmy's office. Vincenzo was incredibly nervous; he was quiet and beside himself. I remember thinking to myself, Please, *God, if this is where we are supposed to be, give me a sign.* At this time, my husband was not entirely excited about holistic medicine, but no matter what, he would try anything to help save his son. I was told to go in with an open mind and that is what we did. I carried my blue composition book with all of Vinny's milestones, and setbacks, and Jimmy just listened. He did not make me feel crazy, and he certainly did not think what happened to Vinny was considered "normal." What he explained to us is that Vinny was affected by heavy metals, not just from vaccines but also from what was in our food. He proceeded to perform a muscle response test with my husband holding Vinny and it was by far the most interesting test I ever witnessed in my life.

The results were hard to hear and confirmed my biggest fear and unfortunately, Vinny was very much affected by this vaccine. I was unaware that the combination vaccines tend to carry more metals than others. I was also unaware that some pediatricians refrain from using combination vaccines due to neurological side effects. I am also learning that many pediatricians offer single-dose MMR to avoid adverse reactions or seizures. You live and learn as a parent, and this was a hard lesson for us that day. There is no one else to blame when we are the parents making decisions for our children who are too young to make those decisions themselves. The organs affected mostly by his vaccine injury were the stomach, liver, and brain. Three vital organs that he needs to thrive were contaminated with metals and toxins. By the time it affected his brain, he was already disconnected from his mother, the mother who carried him for nine months. Jimmy's exact words were, "It is similar to Vinny putting his finger in the electrical socket, setting his brain on fire." That is what my fifteen-month-old went through that night. It makes me feel like the worst mother in the world. I realized as a mother that it was my due diligence to research what exactly is in the vaccines and how we can be more careful moving forward.

That evening, we were given specific instructions to make this transition and healing work. We had to remove all environmental toxins from the home, follow organic diet, and give the supplements to Vinny daily without skipping a dose. I had to think about how I will be able to administer the supplements. Would he take them willingly?

The supplements we were given were to heal the brain, stomach, and liver. Two of the supplements were needed to be given with droppers and the third was a spray for his mouth, and that was the start of his journey. We left the office feeling hopeful and grateful. On our way home, I remember praying to God and hoping that my baby would find his way back to me. That night, we distributed the meds; he opened his mouth willingly for the first supplement but closed his mouth for the second. We gave it sometime and then offered his detox body spray. He did give us a hard time because he was not understanding what was going on, and like I said, it is extremely hard to communicate with a nonverbal child. I told him that we love him and that we will make sure he gets better. I was not giving up on my baby. I was not accepting his drastic change when he was completely fine before the reaction. At this point, we were desperate to try anything and I knew in my heart, this was supposed to be part of his journey.

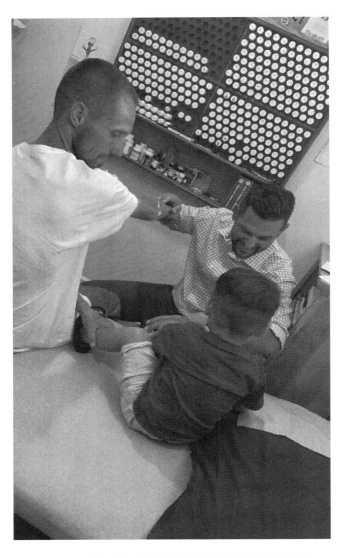

HEALING APPOINTMENT WITH JIMMY
SCARINGI, BRAD, AND VINNY

CHAPTER 9:

# The Start of Healing

The very next evening, Vinny took his supplements without a fuss, and we were astonished by this. Hepatic-Tone has a ridiculously strong taste and smell but my baby did not care. When it was time for his detox spray, he opened his mouth willingly and let us spray his mouth without a problem. On the third day of detox, we noticed a huge change in Vinny. We were scheduled for speech therapy and usually, this was a huge struggle. He did not want to have his sessions over Zoom; he did not understand what we were trying to accomplish and as soon as he saw me reach for the iPad to connect to his therapist, he would throw a tantrum or have a breathing spell. Well, this day that did not happen. I lifted Vinny to put him in his high chair and he did not give me a problem. I proceeded to turn on the iPad and he was still quiet. For a while, his therapist wanted Vinny to learn and attempt to complete a puzzle. The puzzle we attempted was a shape Winnie the Pooh puzzle. When your kid achieves a milestone, the details will never leave you. I placed the puzzle on the table and he started completing the puzzle. Tears streamed down my face as I watched in disbelief. I could not move; I really could not believe that my child was not only completing the puzzle but was doing so with ease. The only change at this point was the supplements, Vinny's diet was already under control, so we knew this milestone was due to the start of his treatment plan.

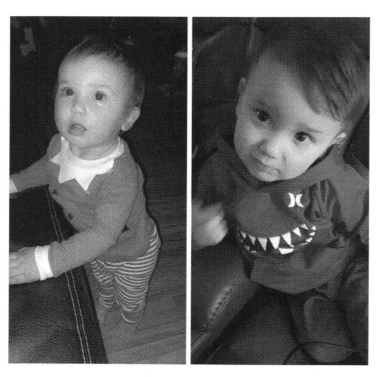

WITH DAYS OF DETOX, HIS SKIN COLOR CAME BACK AND SO DID HIS EYE CONTACT.

One huge red flag we noticed since his reaction was Vinny's sleep pattern. This is also a sign of autism. I was told by the developmental pediatrician that children with ADHD and autism lack melatonin, which in turn prevents them from getting adequate sleep. Vinny went from sleeping and taking naps to not napping and getting up every three hours at the age of two. I was so delusional from not sleeping and getting up with my newborn that I did not realize how stressed and exhausted I was. I never told anyone I needed help, or that I was struggling, and instead, my husband did what we had to do to help our son. On 12/31/20, Vinny slept through the night and slept in until 11:00 a.m. I woke up at 3:00 am to see if he was ready to get up, and nope, he was sleeping like an angel. Again, the only thing we changed at the time was starting the supplements. I remember checking on him multiple times and I could not believe how peaceful our little boy was.

When Vinny woke up that day, he seemed different. Vinny seemed calm, composed, and collected. His body was craving sleep, and finally, he got what he needed. We proceeded to mat time and that is when I started to realize Vinny was changing. Mat time is when Vinny and myself play in the playroom on a mat and complete skill building activities. That day during mat time, I pulled out the same shape puzzle and this kid completed the puzzle even faster than yesterday and he even acknowledged his brother. Prior to this, he could not put two Legos together after his reaction. One of the hardest things to go through was watching your infant surpass your toddler and your toddler not understanding what symbolic play was, or for me, it was the fact that Vinny did not even know how to play with his brother. That evening after his bath, we were looking for the detox spray to give him, and guess where it was? My son was holding the bottle of spray, trying to take the cap off with his teeth. You can say whatever you want but the truth of the matter is that Vinny knew this was helping, and he knew this was a part of his plan. Vincenzo is a special boy serving a higher purpose.

As the days progressed, Vinny was reaching more milestones. Vincenzo was continuing to sit for the speech therapy and would continue to keep eye contact with his therapist. Day four into detox, and Vinny waved bye to his daddy and said bye-bye. My husband ran up to him and hugged him so tight, he said, "That's right, buddy! Bye-bye." Prior to detox, Vinny would have a breathing spell every morning my husband left for work. It was gut wrenching for both of us.

I am telling you, going through a process like this will humble you. One thing is for sure, we will never take our ability to speak for granted. On day five of detox, Vinny demonstrated pretend play. I will never forget this day. It was early in the morning, and I was drinking my coffee and Vinny was over by his kitchen playset. He never really went by the kitchen set because he did not know what to do or how to play with everything. Well, day five of detox changed that for my son. He proceeded to put a piece of food into the pot, took a spoon, and tried to stir it. As I was watching this unfold, I realized this would be something great to record. I grabbed my phone so I could show his therapist and his pediatrician. As I was recording, he continued to take the spoon and put it up to his lips, and I kid you not, he said, "Yum, yum." In two days, my child had said more words than he had since his setback. As a mother, you cannot help but blame yourself for that setback. However, moving forward, the best is yet to come. On day eight, Vinny was able to complete two puzzles and counted to three. You got that right; my boy counted to three!

Another huge accomplishment for Vinny was socialization. For the longest time, Vinny did not want other family members to be around him or in his personal space. He was just afraid of everyone and lost in his own little world. When we were visiting my in-laws, Vinny was able to play with his little cousin Baylie. I could not believe my eyes. They were pushing a toy car back in forth, and he was fully engaged. They have a special connection to this day. Vinny is fully aware of who has patience for him and who does not. Autistic children can feel when someone does not have patience for them.

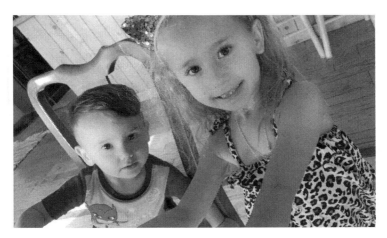

**VINNY AND BAYLIE. HIS ABILITY TO MAKE EYE CONTACT WAS RESTORED.**

However, with every up, there is always down. By day twenty-eight of detox, I caught my son chewing on a penny. I almost had a heart attack. I immediately thought he was going to choke. I kneeled and said, "Vinny, please spit that out right now." He looked at me and thankfully spit the penny out. I did not know what was going on and why the change after he was doing so well; however, with learning so much from Jimmy, I realized that I had to bring this to his attention. He informed me that this was not anything bad that Vinny was displaying but a sign that he is detoxing and may be lacking something. We brought Vinny in; Jimmy adjusted a few things and made sure we left with our supplements. Jimmy could not believe how quickly Vinny was progressing. That night, Vinny detoxed greatly, and the reason I know that was that he was sleeping right next to me and he was surrounded by a puddle of sweat that smelled like metal. As a mother, I cannot explain how I felt that night because it was something I did not want to believe. How did metal get inside of my baby? Jimmy would always say when Vinny would go through a heavy detox to watch out for big milestones. He was right, as always. The very next day, Vinny brought me milk from the fridge, and I looked at him and asked, "Do you want milk? " Vinny responded, "Yes." I started screaming while jumping up and down and held Vinny so tight and said, "I'm proud of you, baby."

As the months progressed, Vinny was able to recite short songs that he would watch on Cocomelon and play with his baby brother without any issues. He began saying, "Mama," and my heart was completely full. For two years, I had been waiting to hear that word. I just remember holding him so tight and saying, "I'm so proud of you, baby. Yes, I'm Mommy!" The biggest accomplishment was his ability to make it through a speech session without a breakdown. His speech pathologist was so blown away by Vinny's progress. He was able to watch her and take it all in.

By April 2021, Vinny was starting to stim more. When Vinny would stim, he would run back and forth multiple times until he wanted to stop. Again, I did not expect his autism to disappear, but I would get concerned when it would happen just because there were now so many more good days than bad. I swear, the hardest part of being a special-needs mother is watching your child go through something and not knowing how you can help them. As the days went on and supplements increased, more words were forming. I will never forget April 13th, 2021. On a messaging app Snapchat, there are many silly filters that can be applied to your photos. On my birthday, I put the birthday one on, and Vinny was sitting next to me. Suddenly, Vinny blurted out, "Happy birthday!" I could not believe my ears just heard my baby say happy birthday. Luckily, I recorded all of this on phone, so I will have it forever. It was the best birthday gift I could have ever received. I highly suggest that when you are going through something with your child, document absolutely everything, and then when they reach certain milestones, you will be able to treasure the memories and work toward achieving what they lack at their age.

Around the end of April, we increased the quantity of detox spray to six sprays at bedtime. On April 23rd, Vinny went to the fridge, opened it up, took out a yogurt, proceeded to walk towards the silverware drawer, took out a spoon, and proceeded to his chair. He finished eating the yogurt until it was gone and then proceeded to the garbage can to throw out his container. I was astonished. He completed all the steps, which is not common with ASD and his age with a fresh diagnosis. Of course, I had to email Jimmy right away and make him aware of every big milestone like this. He said, "Just you wait; there is more to come," and boy was he right!

With May approaching the next day, Jimmy advised us that we are now able to take detox up a notch and place Vinny on an HM-ET Binder capsule daily. At this point, he was on the level of detox that an adult would be taking, and Vinny was two. I was sitting here thinking, "Oh my gosh, it is one thing for Vinny to crave the detox spray, but he is two years old. How am I going to figure this out?" We have come so far with detox, and I was nervous this will disrupt the routine. I always ask God for guidance, whether it is aloud or to myself; I know he will always show me the way. He suggested we could try to open the capsule and add to a smoothie or some type of drink so that he would not be able to figure out it was in there. The next day, we placed the capsule into his milk cup and it turned his milk black. I felt like a failure, thinking he was not going to drink this, no way. He did drink some but would not finish the cup. It was a bright early morning, and we also had speech therapy session later. Now leading up to this day, Vinny was doing great with speech, improving a lot in terms of maintaining eye contact, and sitting still. This morning, that did not happen; instead, he started screaming and hitting himself in the head, and I had to end the session right away. I took him upstairs and I lay down with him. I told him everything was going to be okay and that each day the supplement will be easier to take. This is what I mean about the journey not being an easy one. My child has gone through more detox than most adults can tolerate and the worst thing is that he cannot communicate his pain to me. I have watched him progress in front of my eyes, but I have also witnessed the downfalls. The best thing about Jimmy is that he makes all his patients a priority. He told me to call the office or email at any given time and he will get right back to me. I proceeded to let him know what happened and he said it was signaling that the binder was working and that it was its way of pulling metal out of his body that was still trapped inside. He told me this would not be easy, and I might witness more of that, but he also told to pay attention the next day from having the episode. I had a conversation with my husband and I asked if we should continue with the binder. What I witnessed made me sad, upset, and concerned. Brad said, "Why don't we give it a little more time and make a decision then?" So that is what we did—continued and hoped for the best.

On May 14th, Vinny woke up saying hello. My heart was so full, and we made it downstairs to make breakfast. Vinny came up to me and gave me a high five. I honestly could not believe this, especially with having such a strong episode the day before. I noticed Vinny was sitting by himself, playing with a phone, and he put it up to his ear and said, "Hello." From Vinny putting two and two together and demonstrating pretend play, all I can say is Jimmy was right to say big things would happen the next day. The morning of May 14th, we realized the milk idea did not turn out great, so we had to produce a plan B. After much brainstorming, we decided on putting the capsule in five milliliters of water and drawing it up in a syringe. I will tell you this, that binder has stained my hands, my clothes, and even my sink, so imagine how potent this is. It smells terrible, looks terrible, and all I kept thinking was, *Please,*

*God, let this be the way.* I approached Vinny and said, "Ok, buddy, let us take your supplements." This kid opened his mouth and let me push the supplement through the syringe into his mouth! He did not spit it out. His teeth were black from the stain of the supplement, and all my baby did was smile. I said, "Yeah, buddy, we are so damn proud of you." This showed me here that my son is resilient, he is strong, and most importantly he is my warrior.

On May 17th, however, I observed something very strange. I discovered Vinny was chewing on a penny again. Of course, I phoned Jimmy's office, and he said the binder might be pulling out some of his nutrients, so we needed to add some CT-Minerals to mix. The CT-Minerals were also in drops form, and Jimmy said Vinny probably wouldn't like it directly into his mouth but maybe in water. I approached Vinny with the dropper, and he just opened his mouth like a baby bird and took the CT-Minerals. Now I do not know how your journey will be, but what I can say for Vinny is that he knew the supplements were helping, and he trusted the process. Jimmy was stunned to find out that Vinny was able to tolerate the HM-ET Binder in barely diluted liquid form. After he mentioned that, I realized Vinny was a healer himself. I agreed to the 120 days of HM-ET and continued the process.

On May 20th, I was upset. Vinny was getting his diaper changed and my son's diaper reeked of metals. This was an extremely hard day for me as a mother, again taking me back to self-blame for not researching the combination vaccine that did this to my son. Why wouldn't have I researched about what were putting inside my child or the risk of my child becoming neurologically affected from an adverse reaction? Every child is genetically different and, therefore, vaccine reactions do not affect every single child; however, it affected mine. By May 22nd, Vinny was counting to five and using his fingers, and soon, the first day of the Binder felt like a distant memory and just part of the routine. Stimming became nonexistent and Vinny was even helping wash his brother's hair in the shower! Again, this was achieved with only sixteen days on the Binder, and so many more accomplishments were yet to come. The biggest milestone was that Vinny was finally able to acknowledge his baby brother and show him love and affection.

We entered June with Vinny taking off his diaper, going into the bathroom, and sitting on the potty chair by himself. This was with no direction at all; he did this all on his own. Now when he was twelve months old, he sat on the potty chair by himself and even did a little tinkle, but by the time he was fifteen months old, regression took this habit away. On June 15th, I tried something I never thought I could do. I was going to cut my son's hair. Before learning how to cut his hair, we had a hairdresser who tried hard with him, but it was honestly torturous for both. Vinny would cover ears and hyperventilate and eventually walk around with a crazy haircut. My mother was a hairdresser when we were younger, so I figured was in the middle of detox, I would try taking him to my mother's house. Vinny moved around a little bit but did okay; again, this was only with scissors. By the time I got home, I said, "Okay, Ang, you can do this; get the clippers out of the box, and cut your son's hair." The top was all set, so it was just up to me to buzz the sides and the back. I approached Vinny with the clippers and said, "I want you to hold these in your hands." He held the clippers in his hand and I then turned them on—instead of crying, he started laughing. I also must include that, after that episode, I did end up finding semi-quiet clippers that are available on Amazon. I told him, "Mommy is going to cut your hair. Is that okay?" He smiled, and I just started buzzing his hair. It is so insane how I found the courage to do this but when you are a special-needs child's parent, you will do anything to try and make any situation less stressful for your child. I had to make sure I was as courageous as my child.

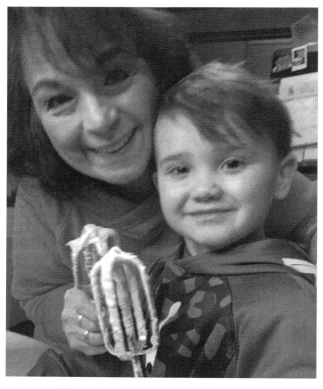

**VINCENZO AND NANA.**
**HE LOVES BAKING COOKIES WITH NANA!**

One thing Vinny loved was his power wheels. On his first birthday, we had bought him a power wheels, and he and his big brother had used up the battery and had so much fun. Fast forward to the regression, and he would scream, run in circles, and cover ears when we would try to get him to ride his once-favorite power wheel. On June 18th, we were sitting in the yard as a family, and Vinny got into the power wheels and started driving around. We could not believe our eyes and just kept chanting, "Go, Vinny; go, Vinny, go!" A few days later, he was whipping around in the power wheels driving like an all-star. Vinny did not drive or bump into anything. It was astonishing to watch, especially with my older son not being able to do that at age two.

On June 25th, I had the biggest pit in my stomach. June 25th was a game-changer, and I will tell you why. The day we went to Robert Warner Institute, we were given instructions by the doctor. The instructions would be sent for Vinny's EEG, blood work, MRI of the brain, and consultation with a geneticist. The reason I was so upset was that if we were to find out this is genetic autism then it would affect his life forever as well as his offspring. I remember Vinny being such a good boy that day; he sat in the waiting room right on my lap and just looked around. When they called his name, he smiled and we proceeded into the exam room. When the doctor came in, she said hello to Vinny and he said hi. Right then and there, she was blown away by his eye contact and his response to her, as she was not expecting that with the diagnosis and evaluations that were performed on him. When the doctor approached the exam table, Vinny grabbed her stethoscope, put it on his chest, and took a few deep breaths. She then took the tongue depressor and asked Vinny what she should do with this and he took the tongue depressor and placed it in his mouth. The doctor looked over to me and smiled, and tears poured down my face. Again, I could not believe my eyes. She finished the exam, looked at me, and said Vinny's Autism is not genetic. She also stated Vinny would not be progressing at a rapid speed if it were genetic autism. She also reiterated that the brain MRI, the blood work, and any other planned testing may be canceled. She finished the visit by saying, "You will not have to come back here and we hope and pray for the best for Vincenzo." We proceeded to check out and the secretary asked when we're coming back, and I did not mean to shout, but I said with excitement, "We do not have to come back!"

Once I buckled him in his car seat, I got into the driver's seat and tears poured down my face and I said, "Thank you, thank you, God, thank you for this miracle." I immediately called my husband and told him the news, and he was so overjoyed. By the end of June, my son was counting to ten and able to name all his primary colors.

With July approaching, we were concerned with the 4th of July. Previous 4th of July, Vinny did not do well. Vinny covered his ears and screamed the entire time, as well as he was suffering from multiple breathing spells. We planned to leave before the fireworks, but it was also unfortunate that my other two children would miss watching them because of Vinny's past episode. However, when you have a child with a disability, you stick together and do the needful. As nighttime approached, we pulled out the double stroller, set Vinny up with his tablet and milk cup, and hoped for the best. As the fireworks started going off, we looked over to Vinny and he was pointing at the firework with the biggest smile on his face. He ended up falling asleep during the fireworks and we then headed home. We are so proud of Vinny; he just keeps on surprising us and making up the proudest parents.

Around the middle of July, Vinny was not himself. He was very pale, and as the day went on, he started crying in pain, and I could not figure out what was wrong. He then started slapping his head and I immediately called our healer. He explained that he had been on the Binder for over a month and it was doing its job. He also said to watch out for any new words that he would say in the next few days. The very next day, my child said, "Be happy" and "I don't care." Now grant it, he learned that phrase from his older brother; I was still happy to hear his little voice. As always, he was right and we just kept trusting the process. By end of July to early August, his vocabulary was increased up to thirty words!

As Vinny's 3rd birthday approached, I could not believe the milestones my baby hit: the fact that people could sing happy birthday to him and he did not cover his ears or run away was so fulfilling. Any time we would sing happy birthday to anyone we would take Vinny out of the room because he would go into sensory overload. It was heartbreaking to watch, especially when his older brother turned seven. We were outside, and Vinny just started screaming, covering ears, and we had to take him away to give him a break. I saw the pain in my older son's eyes because he did not fully understand what was going on here, which we would not expect him to at such a young age. For Vinny's third birthday, we took him to his favorite cabin and boy did we have a blast! He let his cousins play with him and run after him; it was a turning point for our boy. I could barely keep my tears in just so amazed by him and how long he had been into detox at this point. After much thought, I was ready to have Vinny evaluated for preschool and take therapies up a notch. Now that he was three; I brought Vinny into Aspire Center for Learning to have him evaluated for school services.

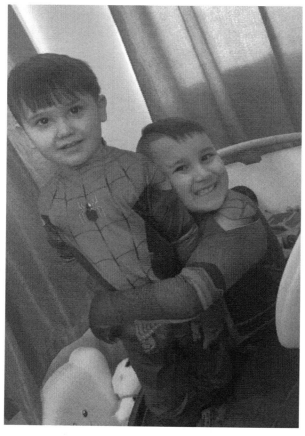

**HE LOVES HIS BIG BROTHER**

# CHAPTER 10:

# Preparation for the First Day of School

My son was diagnosed with autism during the peak period of the pandemic. Therefore, his therapy was extremely limited and consisted of teletherapy or maybe therapy in the backyard if the county allowed that. I remember chasing him around the room with my iPad and trying to get him to sit still while taking care of my infant and homeschooling my oldest. The amount of pressure I was under as a stay-at-home mom was unreal. I was breaking at the seams and this was only the beginning. How could special-needs services be available based on what was going on with the pandemic? Also, if masks were effective then why couldn't he have in-person services? I was done driving myself mad with something that I could not control. The only thing I could control was making sure Vinny was getting the appropriate services, whether it was at home or school.

In preparation for Vinny's Committee Preschool Special Education meeting, we were to have him evaluated by specialists to see which therapies he would qualify for preschool. The therapist called me the night before to let me know when we're doing our evaluation. The school was going to have a practice fire drill. Normally this would send a child into sensory overload. Again, the therapist was going over his evaluations from his developmental pediatrician who performed an evaluation in person on Vinny back in December.

When we arrived in the parking lot, I told Vinny that no matter what the outcome was, I was and will always be super proud of him for being so brave and going through all this testing along with his detox. It just demonstrates how resilient this little boy is. He never gives up. We approached the school and, of course, everybody wore a mask and the teacher approached my son with a thermometer. I was shocked that Vinny just stood there and let them do what they needed to do and then we continued to the classroom. As we proceeded to the classroom, I told Vinny to sit down, and he listened. The therapist was blown away by his eye contact and said, "Wow, I am overly impressed with him already." She then began to work on puzzles with Vinny and he was just cruising right through them. She also presented farm animal toys and he made the sounds for each farm animal and started lining them up. Now when she asked him to point to certain things, he did struggle with that but she even said that some children his age still do not do that. Again, Vinny was only 2.5 years old at the time.

In the middle of the evaluation, the fire bell started ringing and my heart started beating faster because I was not sure what was going to happen. Was Vinny going to have a breathing spell? Was Vinny going to cover ears? Was Vinny going to flip out? As a special-needs mother, you are never prepared for an outburst; however, we were going to see today what would happen. I looked at him and said, "Come on with Mommy. I am going to carry you outside." As I started walking, he clutched onto me and was looking around. So far, he did not cover his ears. As we approached outside and stood in a single file line, Vinny was just looking around and smiling at everybody. It was like he was ignoring what was going on and the fire drill was not even a bother to him. To me, the situation appeared crazy because sensory overload is something that would set him off. The therapist was so shocked and said, "I am so proud of you, Vinny. You are being such a good boy." When the fire drill was over, we proceeded back into the school to finish the evaluation. I was also surprised he wanted to go back into the school willingly.

Once the evaluation was finished, the therapist looked at me and said, "Well, Vinny, we are going to qualify you for speech therapy." I looked at her and I asked, "Are you sure that is all you think that he needs?" And she said, "Absolutely." She explained that Vinny displays high functioning autism, but she was also confused about the significant change from the date of diagnosis to current. At this point, we were seven months into detox and diagnosis. She stated she had never in her career witnessed a turn around like Vinny's. Normally for a child to change that significantly is from intensive therapies that are back-to-back in person multiple days a week. She said, "What I can say for you as his mother is keep doing what you are doing, I am very proud of you and your little guy is going to change the autism world for the good." She told me to keep telling his story and that more kids deserve a chance like him.

I am telling you from start to finish, God lined up nothing but positive people in this journey for Vinny. Everyone supported him; no one thought what we were doing with Vinny was crazy. All I ever heard was "Keep going," "Good work," and "What is the name of your holistic practitioner?" One thing you will have to understand is that people are so quick to judge you with the decisions that you make instead of just supporting you and seeing what the outcome will be. At the end of the day, Vinny is our son and what we do with him is our business and no one else's. As I mentioned previously in this book, do what you need to do for yourself and your family and do not ever let anybody influence your opinion. You must realize the people who are wanting to ruin your journey are not the ones taking care of your child. They do not see what you go through behind closed doors; they have no idea what it is like to have a special-needs child.

On July 22nd, 2021, we had Vinny's CPSE meeting, which of course was done virtually due to the ongoing pandemic. It was an emotional day and a huge turning point for both of us, and I will tell you why. The people who joined the meeting were the speech pathologist who was working with Vinny and the chairperson of the district for special needs to assist with figuring out what services Vinny would qualify for, and which educational environment would help him thrive most. Many children freshly diagnosed with moderate autism do not end up in integrated preschool classrooms. The children who are more severe require more intensive therapies. Everyone was able to speak at the meeting, and when it was my turn, I told them that this had been very rough on my child without getting services and only having thirty minutes of virtual speech; it was not fair to him and he deserved more. He did not ask for this to happen to him and it happened, and we needed to do right by him. Once I was done speaking, the chairperson said, "After reviewing Vincenzo's evaluations and speaking with you and a speech pathologist, I recommend Vinny to attend an integrated preschool with speech therapy three days a week at thirty minutes a day." I said, "Oh, wait a second, so my son is going to be in an integrated preschool? I thought he was going to be in a special-needs setting since he has special needs." She said, "I will have to disagree with you there; he is going to thrive in an integrated preschool and in fact I think if you put him in a special-needs setting, it will be overwhelming for him and could set him back." I took a deep breath and I said, "Thank you."

When I hung up the phone, tears were running down my cheeks and I just looked at Vinny and said, "You did it, buddy! You are thriving so much and every single person that evaluates you sees it." From the geneticist to the therapists evaluating him, everyone saw what me and my husband saw. Sometimes we would have self-doubt and question ourselves if we were the only ones seeing this drastic change in Vinny. After all, we are his parents. But the proof is in my son.

# CHAPTER 11

# Vincenzo's First Day of Preschool

Words cannot describe the anxiety that we carried on Vinny's first day of preschool. The night before school, I could not sleep, my husband could not sleep, and there was just a nervous feeling that surrounded both of us. I kept overanalyzing the entire situation and everything that could go wrong. Here my son was three years old and just turned three in August, yet starting school full-time, and Vinny at this point could not communicate his needs. So now I thought to myself, *What if he cannot tell his teacher that he is upset? Or that he misses his mother? Or that the stimulation is too much? Or what if he gets too hot and needs his sweater off? Or maybe he will need to go to the bathroom and he cannot vocalize anything?* I think the absolute worst thing out of everything was the fact that he would not be able to see his teacher's or aide's faces because they were covered with a mask. So now my biggest fear and my biggest concern would be his interaction with a teacher, as he could not see her mouth move. He already had trouble communicating and now he could not even view emotion on someone's face. I also felt bad for the educators and speech pathologists who had to wear the masks, knowing the children they were talking to were non-verbal and could not see their mouth move.

October 13th, 2021, was Vinny's first day of preschool. I made sure I packed him an awesome lunch, with all his food items in separate containers because Vinny prefers his food that way. I will never forget making shapes of ghosts out of organic turkey and bats out of cheese to get him smiling at lunch time. I made sure his breakfast was perfect too. He prefers pancakes in the shapes of silver dollars and they cannot be cut up. Once his elaborate lunch was made, we packed him up and took him to his first day of school. The hardest part of this day was speaking to the teachers, as we could not see their mouths move, and here I was trying to let them know that masks were new to Vinny and he might be a little frightened. Everything I was worried about now had come true! They took Vinny's hand and led him into the building and they would not let us come into the building. According to the COVID-19 policies, we were not able to walk him into the classroom. As they pulled Vinny away, he started screaming. He was so hysterical, and that image of him will never leave my head.

Of course, I thought fighting for him to not be masked was the hardest thing we would face but I was completely wrong. I even had to fight for this kid to attend preschool because again they wanted an updated MMRV, and that will never happen. Instead, we asked for a script from his pediatrician for titer labs, and long behold, Vinny had positive immunity to MMRV and will never need another vaccine. Yes, you have the right to ask for that as a parent. Do not be afraid to ask for what you need for your child to make sure they will never have an adverse reaction again. For me, vaccines are not the key to perfect health and if it can neurologically change your child or make them have a seizure, I will avoid it at all costs. Yes, it does not happen to every child, but it happened to my child and I will never let that happen again. On December 14th, 2020, I took Vincenzo to outpatient laboratory in our local town. A few days later, I was informed that my son had positive immunity for measles, mumps, rubella, and varicella. Vincenzo no longer needs that vaccine ever again.

| Events | 12/14/2020 12:57 |
|---|---|
| **VIRAL TESTING**   Back to Top | |
| Rubella Virus Ab IgG | 115.4 unit/mL |
| Varicella Virus Ab IgG | NA 1.25 index |
| Rubeola Virus Ab IgG Quantitative Test | NA 4.25 index |
| Rubeola Virus Ab IgG Interp Test | Positive |
| Varicella Virus Ab IgG Interp | Positive |
| **RCDELIVERYRECORDSOURCE**   Back to Top | |
| Rubella Virus Ab IgG | 115.4 unit/mL |

VINCENZO'S LAB RESULTS

Once they walked Vincenzo into the building, I ran back into my truck and started sobbing. Part of me wanted to run back in and get my baby and tell him it would be okay. The other part of me thought I was being a helicopter parent and that how would my child learn to survive in this world if I sheltered him from everything. Would I be setting him back? But what about the trauma? The trauma my son endured when they pulled him away from me, for the first time and he left with strangers, with masks on? Even if they were great, smart educators, how would he know; he could not see their faces? Would Vinny be anxious or was he biting his nails? I remember walking my oldest into his first day of kindergarten and it was such a different experience. I was able to walk my son into his class; we hung his jacket and bookbag in his cubby and then took photos at his desk. I gave him a big kiss and told him I would be back later to pick him up. My child without a disability knew and understood I was coming back to get him. Now fast forward to my special-needs child, who does not understand any of that and even if he did, he was still terrified. Again, he was pulled out of my arms by women with masks on and I could not go with him. Sounds traumatic to me but who am I? Just another special-needs mother who is fighting and advocating for her child! Vinny and I are very connected. I feel what he feels, and it has been this way since the start of his detox. I know exactly how he felt this very day and all I continued to do was pray and hope that God would always protect him and be his voice and advocate when Mommy and Daddy are not around.

On October 14th, Vinny attended his second day of preschool. My husband and I decided that he would do drop-off and I would do pick-up. When my husband approached the doors, Vincenzo seemed okay but it was when his teacher touched his hand that all hell broke loose. Vinny was so hysterical, and my husband demanded to enter the building and settle down his hysterical special-needs child who could not communicate his needs. He was never taking "no" for an answer. Remember, you're fighting your children's fight, and you must never stop fighting. It was then when I realized what a powerful force we have become. My husband has not skipped a beat with Vinny. He is involved with all his care, detox, paperwork, and whatever else comes our way. It is not that we want to shelter our son, but come on, he is recovering from a vaccine injury, and because of that injury, he cannot speak. We get extremely mad at the world and what it has become. We realized at that moment, by the age of five, Vincenzo will more than likely be pulled from school due to the vaccine requirement. This is a never-ending fight for my son who is a vaccine-injured child.

Regardless, of what the future may hold Vinny is thriving and that is all that matters to us. His preschool is amazing astounding and I am blown away by how compassionate his teachers are. We were nervous about winter break and the ten-day quarantine that would affect him as well as finding out we were losing his teacher, due to certain mandates that were going on. As we all know, children with autism thrive off routine and were not only taking his schooling away for a week but were also permanently changing his educator. The days approaching the end of winter break were hard. We knew the changes were coming and on the morning of January 3rd, 2022, my stomach was in knots. It was a very fulfilled morning, full of laughs, giggles, and dancing to Disney's *Encanto*.

Vinny approached me with his bookbag, and I knew he was ready. My husband took him to school and when he approached drop-off, his mind was blown. Vinny took his new teacher's hand and said, "Bye-bye, Daddy." There were no tears, fussing, fighting, breathing spells, or hesitation. Our son was transforming in front of our eyes and I will spend the rest of my life thanking God for giving our baby a second chance at life. Life is hard enough having a disability, but Vinny has demonstrated his disability will never stop him from living a fulfilled life.

CHAPTER 12:

# Do What's Best for You

I wish I could say Vinny's success is because of multiple therapy sessions booked back-to-back in person but I cannot. I wish I could say it was persistent, back-to-back Applied Behavior Analysis therapy but it is not. All I can say is that we were in the middle of a pandemic with no in-person therapy services available. All we had were virtual sessions once a week for thirty minutes. How was this fair to my son? So, I had to figure out the next best step in healing my child and that was finding our healer, along with an extremely strict organic diet and a set of intuitive, loving parents who will never give up! I have been told by medical professionals in our community that this is the quickest turnaround of ASD symptoms that they have ever witnessed. Again, Vinny's T-score was 50; he was displaying severe symptoms of ASD. T-scores are based on a numerical scale that measures a child's performance, and any number over 38 is considered severe autism.

Diagnosed on 1/8/21, and one year later, it's almost un-detectable because he is no longer displaying symptoms of ASD.

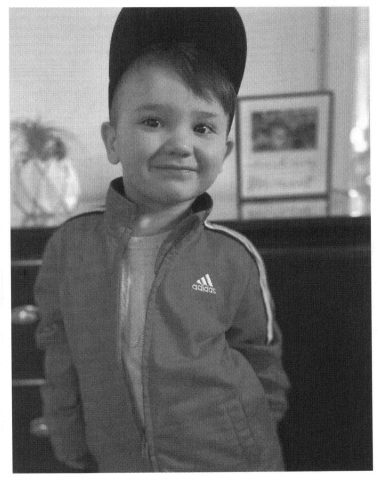

**VINCENZO AGE 3**

No one will ever tell us how to feel, or how to think, when it comes to our children. We learned a valuable lesson here. We are the experts when it comes to our children. No one will say this is not the reason for Vincenzo's regression or that is not the reason for his significant speech delay. Vinny is proof of this story and this miracle. The fact of the matter is that my child was born neurotypical and within hours and days from his fifteen-month wellness visit, he continued to drift further from us. I know family and friends have questioned our beliefs or our decisions, and that's okay. We have no hatred in our hearts from what was spoken about us. At the end of the day, Vincenzo is our child. One thing I can say that is factual is "You will never believe it until it happens to you." You will never care enough until it happens to your child. Stop judging people for them wanting to explore every possible option for their child. The world is so full of judgement that we aren't concentrating on supporting one another and just embracing different styles of parenting. The world is so full of hate, and social media will become the platform for people to take advantage of that. When I first joined social media at the age of thirty-six, I was hoping to connect with other mothers, but that's when I realized how bad social media actually was. I knew I wasn't going to go that route, or make sarcastic videos, trying to prove my point to you. I just knew I had to figure out how to share his story and this is the way we chose to do so.

Again, I reiterate, please do not let anyone disregard you or your child. I cannot fathom the thought of having to go through this without having the footage that I have on my son. I carried a composition notebook everywhere I went because it's just so much information to take in on top of new behaviors developing rapidly. This is how you become the expert, because you have the evidence of your child at every stage of development. Regression is quick and each day without help is damaging to our children.

What I can say from my personal experience is that you must do what is best for your child and your family's situation. I knew as soon as my son had that reaction, we had to prepare ourselves with an open mind to help our child accordingly. At the end of the day, we were willing to go the extra mile to get our son and his speech back. I wanted to hear him say "Mommy" and "I Love You." It is the little things people take for granted daily. We went a full year trying to bring our baby back to us. I wouldn't stop until I see the sparkle in his eye again. We must look at my son Vinny and see the proof in him by his achievements, in such a short period of time.

He, along with many others, will show the world that autism is nothing to be ashamed of or embarrassed of. Autism is absolutely beautiful and I swear they are the most empathetic people. Honestly, the world should be more like them; they have it the hardest and still keep smiling. It's really crazy because Vinny gravitates towards children on the spectrum. Whether he is at school, park, or party, he always ends up finding the special soul amongst the crowds. There is no right or wrong way to treat autism as long as you are doing something to help your child become more sustainable in life.

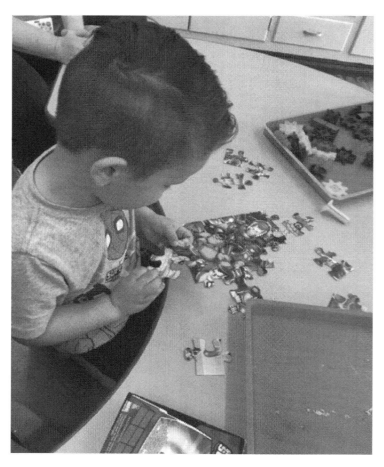

VINCENZO COMPLETING A JIGSAW PUZZLE

# Conclusion

Vinny today can do so many things independently and has reached so many milestones. Vinny can use the bathroom every morning by himself unassisted. He follows using the bathroom with washing his hands and then brushing his teeth. When Vinny attends preschool he is able to use the bathroom unassisted, and he is able to communicate when he needs to use the bathroom. He is now able to dress himself as well as he puts on his jacket, zips it, and puts on his bookbag for school. He also buckles himself in his car seat. He chooses to do all of these things because he now can and wants to demonstrate his independence. Vinny will clean up his mess when he spills something, which is unusual for a kid his age. Vinny will literally run to the counter to grab a paper towel and clean up whatever he spills. He genuinely cares when he disappoints someone, and I cannot believe he can intellectually process all of that. The only reason I say this is because his autism was so severe that I never thought a little over a year he would be able to process that information.

He looks up to his big brother, Luciano, and Luciano is definitely showing him the way. The boys are now tighter than glue. All three of my sons play together, jump on the trampoline, and play on their swing set. I honestly feel this is the biggest accomplishment here—the fact that Vinny can play with his brothers and interact socially with no issues. Vinny is no longer violent; he does not hit anymore; instead, he prefers to hug you. Vinny is able to open the fridge when he is hungry and grab an apple or bell pepper whichever he is in the mood for. He says thank you when someone gives him something and says please if he needs something. He is surpassing milestone after milestone and it's such an amazing feeling as a mother. When Vinny wants milk, he normally brings his cup to me along with the gallon of vanilla almond milk. If he needs water from the filter pitcher in the fridge, he will grab his own cup, go to the fridge, press the button, and never spill a drop while filling the cup! He is also very thoughtful of his baby brother, Alfonso. At times, he will bring him his milk cup and say, "Here, Al," or he will just go up to him and hug him. Sometimes if Al is crying, he will say, "Why are you crying, baby Al?"

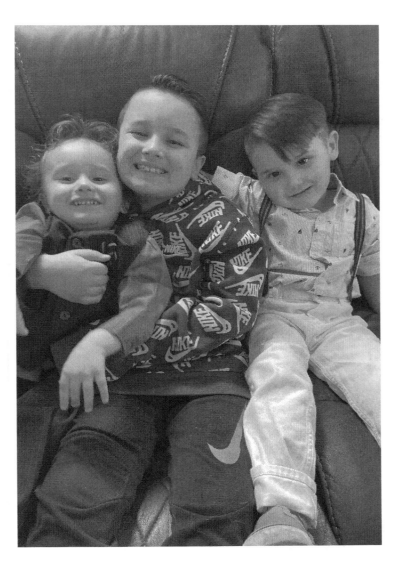

ALFONSO, LUCIANO AND VINCENZO

I will never forget the day I took Vinny go-karting. I was apprehensive to take him go-karting, knowing how loud go-karts are and how fast they go. We approached a go-kart and Vinny was nervous. We proceeded to sit down and buckled ourselves in. As I started to pull off, Vinny covered his ears right away, and I said, "Vinny, don't be scared, buddy; you got this. Grab the steering wheel." I kid you not, that little boy grabbed the steering wheel and away we went. If you could see his smile, you would understand why this was such a big deal for him. I am so glad he can now enjoy things that previously took joy away from him.

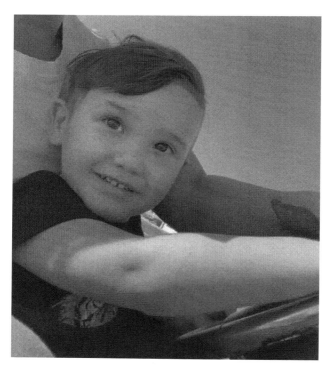

**VINNY DRIVING THE GO-KART.**

His biggest accomplishment thus far was on 3/25/2022. When Vinny was at school, his teacher informed me that my child was able to differentiate between big and small, and when he was asked to circle the correct one, he was able to do that. He was also able to stand in front of his classroom and try to explain the schedule to the class. Of course, all of his words are not perfectly clear but at least we hear his voice. Later that evening, I was sitting with Vinny on my lap and we were reading the book *"Brown Bear, Brown Bear, What Do You See?"* Vinny took the book out of my hands and read the words, "Brown Bear, Brown Bear, What Do You See?" I could not believe what I just heard! My son was trying to read at the age of three, having ASD and freshly diagnosed. As of 4/11/22, my son is able to read the entire book!

What we have witnessed here is a God-given miracle and Vinny having a second chance at life that's not so hard. I am grateful for my husband, who is my rock and my absolute best friend. Without him, we would not have been able to complete this journey. He works a hard physical job to provide for a family of five and he does an exceptional job at it. As you know, health insurance does not cover holistic medicine, so everything we did for Vinny was out of pocket. Vinny did not go one day without a supplement. It takes consistency to make this happen. Detox is one part, but diet, and having a toxin-free home is the other part. Our children have never been this healthy. In one full year, my children have not needed antibiotics or doctor's appointments. We have almost fully healed all of their gut damage. We no longer need fever reducers, and if we do, we choose to treat the fever the way we were taught by Jimmy.

I am eternally grateful for Jimmy and the people who are now family that have connected us. Jimmy has been nothing but kind, genuine, and honest with us from start to finish. He has seen us at our lowest and highest during this journey and has always remained so positive and so pure. He is a God-given angel who can heal, and Vinny is the proof of that. On top of having Jimmy and the Synergy family, Vinny also has an amazing pediatrician who respects our views on vaccinations and provides the upmost care to my boys.

For anyone who is reading this book, I want you to never give up. We understand that the word "autism" means lifelong diagnosis, but it does not define your child. This is just Vinny's story but it does not mean it will not happen with your special-needs child. You may have a faster or slower journey, but it will take dedication and consistency all the way through. Whether it was us bringing our own snacks to a birthday party or going on a vacation, the supplements and diets followed us everywhere. Dedication and consistency are key to success.

I've been asked many times what if someone else goes through what Vinny did and they do not get the same outcome? My response was, "Even if you go through this process and you lose one symptom, or gain one milestone, isn't it all worth it?" I know, to my family, it was worth it. Having the right tools at the right time can produce miracles. Our son is the proof of that.

It was very hard to share this story, and I really hope it can make a difference and help someone else. To all of the specials-needs mothers out there who are continuing to fight for their special-needs children, I have the upmost respect and love for you. I want you to know I see you and hear you, and I respect whatever route you decide take for your child. I also wanted to personally thank everyone who decided to purchase this book and support my son's detox journey. We are forever thankful and grateful; it takes a village.

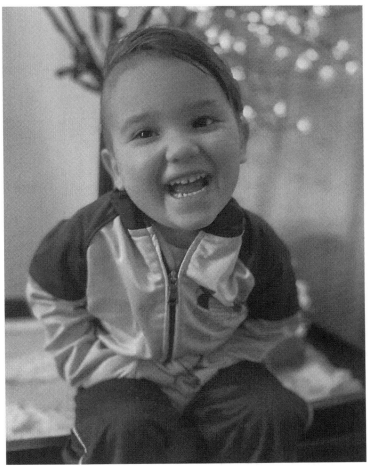

**IT'S THE SMILE FOR ME.**

# About the Author

Angela Acker and her husband Bradley are the proud parents of Vincenzo Roman. Vincenzo was created through love and science, and for that Angela and Bradley are eternally grateful. They always thought the hardest part would be conceiving Vincenzo, but they were wrong. When he was born he was neurotypical, hitting milestones and becoming his own person like all other kids. Then something happened. Suddenly, his light was gone and he drifted far away. Vincenzo was diagnosed with level 2 Moderate Autism. His T-Score was equivalent to 50, demonstrating severe symptoms of ASD. Vinny was now completely nonverbal, ear covering, hurting himself, screaming, falling, mouthing, spinning in circles, breath-holding, hand flapping, and staring off into space. But the worst thing that happened was that he disconnected himself from everyone, but especially Angela.

Angela never wants another parent to go through what her family had to endure. In this highly personal and emotional account of their journey, she tells readers what they did and how much it helped Vincenzo. It was never about who or what to blame for autism, it was all about moving forward. If hearing Vincenzo's story can help just one other child, then sharing their difficult journey will have been worthwhile.

Follow their journey on Facebook at **Angela Lynn | Facebook** and Instagram under **vincenzos_army**

Made in the USA
Columbia, SC
23 December 2023

29378259R00050